Contents

What Exactly is Alzheimer's?

Alzheimer's disease is commonly called dementia. There is no cure for the disease, which worsens as it progresses, and eventually leads to death. It was first described by German psychiatrist and neuropathologist Alois Alzheimer in 1906 and was named after him.

As uncommon as the name of the disease sounds, its prevalence and incidence rates are not. In fact, almost four million people in the United States are affected by this problem. All can be affected, men or women, across all social status and economic position in life.

Alzheimer's is a progressive and degenerative problem under the umbrella of diseases called dementia. It is characterized by disorientation and impaired memory. It is apparently caused by an attack in the brain, affecting one's memory, thinking skills and judgment. Most patients will experience a change in language ability, in the way they use their mental processes and of course their behavior.

While anybody can be affected by this problem, only those that are older than age 65 experience the lagging in their thinking skills. Still, there are some who gets Alzheimer's even when they are just 30 years old but these cases are very rare and can only account for a small percentage of the total number of cases. One out of 10 people over the age 65 has Alzheimer's and nearly half of these patients are over 85 years old. In a national survey conducted in the United States, almost 19 million Americans have one family member who suffers from this dreaded problem.

In addition to old age, family history of dementia can also predispose someone to the disease. This is because Alzheimer's is said to be caused by a problem in the genetic mutations. Still, when you study the cases, Alzheimer's is commonly the result of a host of other factors besides genes. In fact, environmental factors such as hobbies and mental pursuits are things that can help prevent the onset of the problem.

What is difficult with Alzheimer's is the fact that its symptoms are basically the same with ordinary signs of old age. At the beginning, there will be some memory loss. The person with Alzheimer's will also experience confusion and disorientation even with things that they are used to doing. The trick is to make sure that one can recognize what a normal memory loss is against something of Alzheimer's caliber.

Often, there will be a gradual memory loss. They will find it hard to read or to write or to think clearly. After which they will experience a decline in the ability to perform tasks that are already automatic and routinely. Believe it or not, in cases that are already in the terminal stage, the patient may even forget how to brush their teeth or how to use a spoon and fork, something that is really pretty basic with a lot of people.

This is one example of the difference of Alzheimer's from ordinary memory loss. Forgetfulness will not affect tasks that are routinely. There will also be difficulty in learning new things and in memorizing things. Some patients may even forget the language that they are speaking with while others will no longer recognize their family. Personality will change in terms of the way they communicate with other people and the way they behave.

There is actually no change in personality per se but because of the problems in their memory, they may appear aloof and suspicious perhaps because they cannot

3

recognize the people that they know before. Some may even become extremely fearful and passive for the simple fact that they cannot remember you. As the disease worsens, the patient will then become so incapable of taking care of themselves that they will require help even in eating and in sleeping.

Alzheimer's disease is the most common cause of dementia, affecting around 496,000 people in the UK. The term 'dementia' describes a set of symptoms which can include loss of memory, mood changes, and problems with communication and reasoning. These symptoms occur when the brain is damaged by certain diseases and conditions, including Alzheimer's disease. This factsheet outlines the symptoms and risk factors for Alzheimer's disease, and describes what treatments are currently available.

During the course of the disease, protein 'plaques' and 'tangles' develop in the structure of the brain, leading to the death of brain cells. People with Alzheimer's, also have a shortage of some important chemicals in their brain. These chemicals are involved with the transmission of messages within the brain. Alzheimer's is a progressive disease, which means that gradually, over time, more parts of the brain are damaged. As this happens, the symptoms become more severe.

Alzheimer's Basic Information

Unbelievably, one out of ten people over the age of 65 have Alzheimer's disease. In fact, in a recent statistic polls, almost 19 million Americans suffer one way or the other from this dreaded progressive disease. Below is some information that you will find useful about the disease.

What is Alzheimer's disease?

Alzheimer's disease is a degenerative problem characterized by memory loss as well as loss in thinking skills. It is actually part of a constellation of memory and brain problems called dementia. It can lead to behavioral changes, loss of language skills, disorientation, confusion and increasing dependency. Most experts believe that Alzheimer's is caused by a problem in the genetic make-up and is often associated with old age.

What are the signs and symptoms of Alzheimer's disease?

What is however difficult with this problem is the fact that the onset of the disease will often manifest in symptoms often associated with forgetfulness when getting old. What separates this problem though is the fact that people with Alzheimer's will eventually even forget normal routines and simple tasks. For instance, patients with Alzheimer's can forget how to hold a spoon and fork while others will forget how to brush their teeth and take a bath. Believe it or not, some medical experts even say that some even forget hoe to breathe, something which comes quite naturally with a person.

One problem though with this is the fact that one can actually have no way of knowing whether it is ordinary forgetfulness or Alzheimer's when it is just in the initial stages. It can start with ordinary forgetting of names and faces until it progresses to something major that can render the person totally incapacitated.

For many people, detecting the first signs of memory problems in themselves or a loved one brings an immediate fear of Alzheimer's disease. However, most people over 65 experience some level of forgetfulness. It is normal for age-related brain shrinkage to produce changes in processing speed, attention, and short term memory, creating so-called "senior moments." Forgetfulness is merely inconvenient, though, and generally involves unimportant information. Understanding the significance of these age-related changes begins with knowing the difference between what is normal and what is an early symptom of Alzheimer's.

Who are affected by Alzheimer's disease?

Although there are cases of Alzheimer's that affected people in their 30s, most patients are over the age of 65 and a vast majority is over the age of 85. In addition to old age, experts believe that a family history of the same problem or of dementia may predispose someone to the disease. This is because experts pinpoint a defect in the genetic make-up of the person who has Alzheimer's disease.

People who are not much into mental pursuits or work that do not much involve mental strains will also most likely develop the disease compared to people who often stretch their mental muscles. In fact, one of the ways to prevent the onset of dementia is to exercise the brain all the time especially during old age.

Even when one is already retired from work, old people should not forget to still use their minds by engaging in mental pursuits such as reading, answering crossword puzzles and even playing board games.

How do you diagnose Alzheimer's Disease?

As mentioned earlier, it is extremely difficult for a person to differentiate an ordinary case of forgetfulness and dementia at the beginning of the progression. Some of the symptoms of the disease such as slow mental processing and forgetfulness may be attributed to other problems such as thyroid gland problems, reactions to medications that are being taken, and even just a normal aging process.

To really ensure that the problem is indeed Alzheimer's, doctors rule out other possibilities and conduct series of tests. The only way actually to conclusively determine the presence of Alzheimer's is to examine a cross section of the brain tissue when a person is already dead.

Since there is no single definitive medical test for identifying Alzheimer's disease, arriving at the correct diagnosis can take time and patience. The most important step is to assess past and present functioning. Determining classic patterns can not only help your doctor eliminate other causes of Alzheimer's symptoms, but also distinguish Alzheimer's from other forms of dementia. Your doctor will gather family history information, order medical tests, and estimate your memory loss using a variety of assessments. To diagnose Alzheimer's disease from your symptoms, a doctor will look for many aspects like significant memory problems in immediate recall, short-term, or long-term memory.

Significant thinking deficits in at least one of four areas: expressing or comprehending language; identifying familiar objects through the senses; poor coordination, gait, or muscle function; and the executive functions of planning, ordering, and making judgments. Decline severe enough to interfere with relationships and/or work performance. Other causes to be ruled out – to ensure memory and cognitive symptoms are not the result of another medical condition or disease, such as Mild Cognitive Impairment.

Understanding Alzheimer's Better

Alzheimer's information is important for individuals who may be at the first stages of this disease. However, it is also very important for friends, family and caregivers of people with Alzheimer's disease to have enough Alzheimer's information to be able to understand the process of the progression of the disease as well as what to expect and what is the best care and treatment for this.

To understand Alzheimer's more, we need to look at and understand dementia. Dementia is a mental disorder characterized by the loss of cognitive abilities. It is an extremely debilitating disease that afflicts some individuals in their old age. Alzheimer's information shows that Alzheimer's disease is the most common form of this disorder that greatly impairs normal mental operations.

There is no certain prevention or cure for Alzheimer's disease right now but continuous studies and tests are being made toward this endeavor because according to Alzheimer's information, this disease is irreversible. The disease also continues to progress into different stages and symptoms of this worsen over time.

One of the earliest symptoms of Alzheimer's is short term memory loss. It then progresses into a gradual decline of other cognitive abilities. After the disease has progressed further, one may notice a marked change in the sufferer's behavior and at the very last stages of the disease, the individual with Alzheimer's will have to depend on others for simple activities such as eating and mobility.

Alzheimer's information tells us that the course of the disease varies from person to person with a range of five to twenty years. Alzheimer's eventually ends in death due to complications and infections.

Although more and more Alzheimer's information has been collated and researched throughout the years, the progress has been steady but slow. For instance, the Alzheimer's information on what causes the disease is still uncertain. There are some major hypotheses that seem to revolve around two factors: genetic or hereditary and a complex environmental interaction.

Alzheimer's information shows us that it is primarily a disease that affects the brain. It is in the abnormalities in the brain that result in massive atrophy of the brain's neurotransmitters, nerves and neurons. From these stem the malfunctions that begin with short term memory loss to sever impairment to memory and the loss of motor skills and other normal bodily functions.

An abnormally large deposit of protein in the brain causes the massive atrophy. The absolute detection of Alzheimer's can only really be done post mortem through an autopsy where the brain is examined and it shows a significant amount of shrinkage and a smoothening of the usual brain wrinkles.

However, one need not wait for an autopsy to find out whether one is suffering from Alzheimer's disease or not. With modern Alzheimer's information, one can have an 85 % to 90% accuracy in the diagnosis of the disease. No laboratory tests are done.

Instead, there will be some cognitive tests and with a series of exercises and questions that are crossed checked against other possible sources of dementia. These mental tests done to be able to diagnose Alzheimer's help also by letting the physician know at which stage of progression the sufferer may be at.

Individuals with the age of 65 and above are most likely to be at risk of Alzheimer's.

Origins Unknown, the battle with Alzheimer's continues

In 1901, a 51-year-old woman, Auguste D, was admitted to the state asylum in Frankfurt. She was suffering from cognitive and language deficits, auditory hallucinations, delusions, paranoia and aggressive behaviour, and was studied by Alois Alzheimer (1864–1915), a doctor at the hospital.

Alzheimer moved to the Munich medical school in 1903 to work with Emil Kraepelin – one of the foremost German psychiatrists of that era – and when Auguste D died in April 1906, her brain was sent to him for examination. In November of that year, Alzheimer presented Auguste's case at a psychiatry meeting, and he published his talk in 1907.

In 1910, Kraepelin coined the term 'Alzheimer's disease' – a term still used to refer to the most common cause of senile dementia. But had Alzheimer actually discovered a new disease, and was Kraepelin justified in calling it such?

One could trace back the history of Alzheimer's disease from a presentation and lecture made by a German psychiatrist in 1906 during 37th Meeting of Southwest German Psychiatrists held in Tübingen.

When Dr. Alzheimer autopsied the patient's brain, he found thick deposits of neuritic plaques outside and around the nerve cells. He also found a lot of twisted bands of fibers or neurofibrillary tangles inside the nerve cells.

Today, medical specialists need to find the presence of the same plaques and tangles at autopsy in order to have a conclusive diagnosis that Alzheimer's disease indeed caused the disease. And due to this lecture and achievement in research and studies, the medical community has bestowed the honor of naming the disease after Dr. Alzheimer.

However, Dr. Alzheimer's work only signaled the start of years of medical research and studies which could only resolve the mysteries of the disease by so much. Up until now, Alzheimer's disease has still unknown origin and remains to have no cure. At first, the diagnosis of Alzheimer's disease was limited for individuals between the ages of 45-65 since the symptoms of pre-senile dementia due to the histopathologic process are more common and prominent during this age.

However, during the 1970s and early 1980s, the term Alzheimer's disease began to be used to refer to patients of all ages that manifest the same symptoms.

Statistics show that around 350,000 new cases of Alzheimer's disease are being diagnosed each year. It is estimated that by 2050, there are 4.5 million Americans afflicted by the disease. Recent studies have shown that there is an increased risk of contracting and developing Alzheimer's as one grows older.

It has been reported that 5 percent of Americans between the ages of 65 to 74 suffer from Alzheimer's disease. Also, half of those in the 85 years and older age group are more likely to have the disease.

Generics have also been seen as a factor in the development of the disease. Scientists have found out that mutations on chromosomes 9 and 19 have been associated with the later stages of Alzheimer's. However, not everyone that manifests the mutations results to having the disease. Up until now, the relationship between genetics and late-onset Alzheimer's is still a grey area.

Meanwhile, other research have associated trauma as a factor that increases the risk of acquiring the disease. There are also evidences which suggest that lack of exercise increases the risk factor of Alzheimer's. It is important to avoid high blood pressure, high cholesterol, and low levels folate in order to decrease the risk of developing the disease.

There are basically three stages of Alzheimer's disease. Stage 1 or Mild Stage is the early of the disease. At this stage patients become less energetic and will experience slight memory loss. Often times, the symptoms at this stage are either go unnoticed or are ignored as but trivial or normal occurrences.

At Stage 2 or Moderate stage, the patient needs to be assisted in some complicated tasks and memory loss is no highly noticeable. The final stage is the severest stage. Because the disease already progresses too far this point, the patient is unable to perform simple tasks and will lose the ability to walk or eat without help.

Finding out Early On about Alzheimer's

Alzheimer's is an extremely debilitating disease. Presently, there are no known cures or treatment for this irreversible threat to a mature person's mental and personal health. Once a person has been diagnosed with Alzheimer's, the duration and course of the disease will vary from five up to twenty years.

Within the course of the disease, the sufferer will go through a whole range of deterioration from slight short term memory loss to the loss of normal bodily functions that cause complications and infections that then turns into death.

While the prospect of Alzheimer's disease is truly grim, there continues to be steady breakthroughs from experts that help hope persist that eventually, prevention and cure for Alzheimer's may be found. Before that though, there are lot of questions to be answered and the race to find the cure continues.

Despite this, it is important to take note of the early signs of Alzheimer's, for friends loved ones and yourself. Taking note of the early signs of Alzheimer's will help everyone involved prepare and understand all that is entailed in arranging for care and what to expect as the illness progresses.

It is important to be on the lookout for early signs of Alzheimer's if you or someone you care for is nearing the age of 65 or if there is known cases al Alzheimer's in the family.

Below are some early signs of Alzheimer's to look out for.

Downscale

While memory loss is commonly mentioned as the one of the early signs of Alzheimer's, it has been noted that unexplained and sudden weight loss usually occurs within individuals who suffer from Alzheimer's. They have found that the weight loss happens way before any actually memory loss begins.

If you or someone you care about begins to lose weight unexpectedly, consult your doctor for probable cause and if there are no reasons found then you should have tests for Alzheimer's done.

Forgetfulness

The most common early sign of Alzheimer's is the loss of short term memory. More often than not, at the very early stages, this short term memory loss often goes unnoticed so it is important to pay close attention and see if it is normal memory loss or is it an early sign of Alzheimer's.

While everyone will forget something once in a while, but Alzheimer's sufferer never recall back what has been lost. So pay attention for peculiar incidences of short term memory loss that result in the distress, however much slight, in everyday routine.

Disability

Alzheimer's will rob one of the ability to do the things that used to come second nature to them. It is as if the individual with Alzheimer's can no longer remember or are familiar with tasks or actions that used to be part of their everyday routine. Watch out for this telltale sale that is quite an indicator included in the early signs of Alzheimer's disease.

More Changes

Another early sign of Alzheimer's is the increasing problem of communication. Often, people with Alzheimer's will have a difficult time communicating because they begin to lose their ability to handle language. They begin to forget simple words and terms and their sentence construction begin to be difficult to understand.

There can also be a change in behavior or mood that is not normal for the person with Alzheimer's disease. Over and above moodiness, a person with Alzheimer's can switch moods or behavior without reason.

The main reason Alzheimer's disease shortens people's life expectancy is not usually the disease itself, but complications that result from it. As patients become less able to look after themselves, any illnesses they develop, such as an infection, are more likely to rapidly get worse. Caregivers will find it harder and harder to identify complications because the patient becomes progressively less able to tell if he/she is unwell, uncomfortable, or in pain. Pneumonia and pressure ulcers are examples of common complications which may lead to death for people with severe Alzheimer's disease.

Tell Tale Signs of Alzheimer's

Alzheimer's disease is a progressive brain disorder. Its gradual effects on the brain are relentless as a sufferer's memory is progressively destroyed and along with it, the capability to learn, make judgments, and communicate. The disease will eventually make it difficult for the sufferer to even carry out normal daily tasks to the point of total disappearance of any capability.

It is a very difficult circumstance to be in, to watch a family member seemingly "waste away" bit by bit. The sufferer's the struggle to maintain some form of sanity despite the condition is often too much for many relatives to bear that they, sadly, distance themselves from the sufferer instead of giving support.

It really pays to know more about Alzheimer's and better understand the condition lest you find yourself or a member of your family in this type of situation. Knowing the warning signs early on can help you cope up with the disease earlier where there might still be some chance at minimizing the damaging effects of Alzheimer's. Knowing what to look for will not only help you but also your friends or loved ones who might also have the odds against them in developing the said debilitating disease.

It is of the utmost important to understand some of the warning signs of Alzheimer's. While memory loss is reasonable and is an expected symptom of aging, the type of memory loss symptoms of Alzheimer's are significantly greater and are often accompanied or followed by other tell-tale symptoms. People suffering this disease often have difficulty with general cognitive abilities such as communication, thinking, reasoning, comparing, and learning new skills.

Short-term memory is what Alzheimer's disease usually affects first. Sufferers tend to forget family names and even how to perform simple daily tasks. However, long-term memory is somehow attained with Alzheimer's disease where some patients may even retain the ability of remembering events from the past.

Another sign shown by patients suffering from Alzheimer's disease is the gradual loss of verbal communication skills. Instead of speaking up, sufferers will begin to communicate their feelings, preferences and needs through body language and facial expressions more frequently. Perception is another area that can be affected by Alzheimer's disease.

It may be difficult to set up a clear warning sign level as some of the symptoms exhibited by Alzheimer's sufferers might just be a part of normal behavior. Such symptoms may even be related to another ailment entirely. But when you see such signs being exhibited by someone near to you or someone that you know, you should never be quick to rule out Alzheimer's as a possible reason. Here are the ten basic warning signs for Alzheimer's to always look out for:

•Gradual loss of memory

•Difficulty performing simple everyday tasks

•Problems with language

•Disorientation

•Declining judgment

•Inability to perform complex mental tasks

•Misplacing certain everyday items

•Noticeable behavioral changes

•Increased confusion, fear and suspicion

•Loss of initiative

As of the present there are no Alzheimer's treatments that will totally cure, prevent or reverse the onset of the disease or its gradual progression. What doctors can do is try to treat many of the disease symptoms such as loss of memory. The good news is that as new discoveries about the disease are being made, it won't be long before effective Alzheimer's treatments will be made available.

Try to consult with a qualified physician in order to help eliminate some symptoms that might look like true Alzheimer's and to effectively distinguish between the many other causes of dementia, some of which are completely treatable.

What to Look Out For in Alzheimer's

Alzheimer's disease is a slow brain disorder the eats away the brain functions little by little. The disease develops completely between seven to 10 years. As it progresses, the disease affects various brain functions like memory, movement, judgment, abstract reasoning and even one's behavior.

Because of the long development stage of the disease, Alzheimer's has been categorized into three levels which described its progression. These are mild, moderate and severe. These categories defined the disease from early (mild) to middle (moderate) until the final (severe) stages of the disease.

During the early stages of the disease, the symptoms are less noticeable and are often times left unchecked and considered trivial by family members and even the patient themselves. Among the early and classic signs Alzheimer's disease is the gradual loss of short-term memory.

At times, they find to be at lost while performing normal activities. Or they might get disoriented and get lost in places that they have been before. Also, at this stage, people afflicted with the disease may experience lapses of judgment and slight changes in personality. Mood swings and personality changes will start to worsen as the disease progress.

Moreover, attention span is reduced because of the presence of the brain disorder. People with Alzheimer's tend to be less motivated to complete activities or tasks. Furthermore, they become more stubborn and would oppose changes and new challenges set forth before them.

These are the general conditions or symptoms of people with the disease. The symptoms vary from person to person. Moreover, some other symptoms include speech problems, failure to identify or recognize objects, no recalling how to use simple, ordinary things like a pencil, and not remembering to turn off the lights, stove, or even lock doors and windows. As the disease progresses so do the symptoms.

However, if one acquires or notice the presence of some of the symptoms it does not necessarily mean that one has already been afflicted with the disease. Loss of memory for example might be just a normal cause of aging or other normal factors. Memory loss in Alzheimer's is more frequent.

People with the disease will more frequently forget words or names during conversations. And because they become conscious of their forgetfulness, they tend to avoid conversations and would rather keep quiet in order to avoid mistakes and embarrassments. They will then become withdrawn which can cause a myriad of other problems like depression and anti-social behaviors.

Other things that might happen are the discovery of things in odd places. One might find books inside freezers, clothes in dishwasher and even plates in washing machines. People with Alzheimer's will ask questions repeatedly up to the point that it becomes irritating. They can be provoked quite easily and can surprisingly flare up in anger.

Even though no cure has yet been discovered or developed for Alzheimer's, there are ways that have been created to delay the progression of the disease. Earlier symptoms of the disease respond well to various treatments.

Because the rate of progression differs from person to person, severe dementia occurs within five years to a decade after diagnosis. Because of present treatments and medications, some people diagnosed with Alzheimer's can live more than 10 years after diagnosis. Some even live up to 20 years after the initial diagnosis was made.

It is a fact that most people with Alzheimer's don't die of the disease itself, but of infections and other tertiary diseases like pneumonia, or urinary tract infection or complications resulting from concussions.

Stages of Alzheimer's Disease

Medical science has determined a lot of things through the years. It has discovered various diseases and its causes. Unfortunately, there are still a lot of unknowns. Doctors are unable to determine the cause of cancer, the cure for AIDS and even something that called Alzheimer's disease.

Alzheimer's is considered to be a disorder that will affect one's mental and physical state. It normally happens to people 65 years of age and above that can affect anyone regardless of sex.

There are seven known stages for this type of disorder and it only gets worse as time goes by.

In the first stage, the individual and those around will not notice anything wrong. The person may forget a thing or two, which everyone experiences so there is no cause for alarm yet.

During the second stage, the person may already feel something wrong as this memory lapses happen more frequently. Again, there is no need yet to be alarmed because people tend to forget things due to aging.

The third stage is the time when someone can be suspected of having this disease. The person will falter at work or be unable to accomplish some simple tasks and people will take notice of these changes.

In the fourth stage, the individual can no longer handle certain activities and will require the assistance of those around to accomplish it.

The fifth stage is what doctors describe to be moderate Alzheimer's disease. The individual will not only forget other people but also be unable to recall certain facts about oneself. There will also be periods of disorientation.

In the sixth stage better known as moderately severe Alzheimer's, there will already mood swings. The patient may be happy and in the next minute appear hostile to those around. There will also be fecal and urinary incontinence just like a baby who is not yet toilet trained.

The seventh and final stage is called severe Alzheimer's. The individual will not be able to speak much and do anything anymore. The patient will probably just stare into space so there will be times that those around will have to carry and force feed to be able to stay alive.

Alzheimer's disease happens gradually. The only thing people can do is slow down the process before it gets to the succeeding stage by using drugs and giving proper care to the patient.

As the patient's condition gets worse, the person is no longer treated as a human being by merely as a subject with the disorder. This shouldn't be the case given that the individual at point in life accomplished a lot of things and never wanted this to happen in the end.

There are more than four million people in the United States that are diagnosed with this disorder. This number will definitely grow in the years to come as more and more Americans will reach the retirement age.

Those who have family members who are suffering from this disease should learn about the various stages to be able to understand what the patient is going through to give the proper help.

There are books and other information on the web as well as support groups since this disease affects not only the patient but also those who have to live with it.

Alzheimer's, Not Just an Old Man's Disease

Alzheimer's disease, we've all hear of it but do we really understand the disease? According to statistics, there are about 350,000 new cases of Alzheimer's disease diagnosed each year in the United States.

Doing the math, you could have more than 4.5 million Americans by the year 2050 that would be affected by the disease. A grimmer outlook indicates that by 2025, there will be 34 million people worldwide Alzheimer's disease.

Let's tackle the issue step by step. Alzheimer's disease is a known brain disorder that is progressive and irreversible. It is still not known where and how the disorder develops in the human brain neither is there any sure fire cure for the disease. What is known by medical scientists is that the disease attacks slowly.

It takes its time, gnawing slowly at the victims' minds stealing memories and causing deterioration of brain functions. Alzheimer's is a disease that causes irreversible dementia and is always fatal.

It was German psychiatrist Dr. Alois Alzheimer who first identified the disease. At first he noted the disease's symptoms as "amnestic writing disorder," however when later studies were conducted Dr. Alzheimer found out that the symptoms were more than ordinary memory loss. It was far worse.

Dr. Alzheimer found the presence of neurofibrillary tangles and amyloid plaques in the brain. The good doctor presented his findings which were accepted by the medical community. And soon enough, by 1910 the name of the disease was accepted and became known as Alzheimer's disease.

The most common early symptoms of the disease are confusion, being inattentive and have problems with orientation, personality changes, experiencing short-term memory loss, language difficulties and mood swings. Probably the most obvious and striking early symptom of Alzheimer's is loss of short term memory.

At fist the victim will exhibits minor forgetfulness, but as the disease slowly progress he/she will start to forget a lot of things. However, older memories are oftentimes left untouched. Because of this, patients with Alzheimer's will start to be less energetic and spontaneous. As the disease progress, they will have trouble learning new things and reacting on outside stimuli which gets them all confused and causes them to exercise poor judgment. This is considered Stage 1 of the disease.

At Stage 2 the patient will now need assistance in performing complicated tasks. Speech and understanding is evidently slower. At this stage, Alzheimer's victims are already aware that they have the disease which causes a whole lot of problems like depression and restlessness.

At this point, only the distant past can be recalled and recent events are immediately forgotten. Patients will have difficulty telling time, date and where they are.

The final stage is of course the hardest, both for the patient and their family. At Stage 3 the patient will start to lose control of a lot of bodily functions like simple chewing and swallowing. He/she will start getting the needed nutrients through a tube. At Stage 3, the patient will no longer remember basically anyone.

They will lose bowel and bladder control and they will become vulnerable to third party infections and diseases like pneumonia.

Once the patient become bedridden, things will only get worse. Respiratory problems will become more terrible.

It is apparent that the patient will need constant care. At this point, the most one can do is to make sure that the patient stays as comfortable as possible. At the terminal stage, death is inevitable.

Symptoms of Alzheimer's

When word Alzheimer's is mentioned, the first thing that comes to mind is memory loss. This assumption is correct given that the doctors have determined this to be a disorder that usually happens to old folk.

There are many symptoms of Alzheimer's and doctors often associate it with the seven stages. There is no cause of alarm yet in the first two stages since even the smartest people tend to forget things every so often.

The first two stages may last for four years. However, when this happens more frequently, the patient could already be in the third or fourth stage and this is just going to get worse. A simple example could be if the individual is unable to complete a simple task that was easily done in the past like doing some basic arithmetic.

People will definitely notice the changes. This is the reason some family members take shifts watching over the loved one or get a nurse to watch over the person.

The fifth stage is better known as moderate Alzheimer's because aside from not being able to recall names or do things without assistance, the individual will become disoriented and may at times get lost.

One precaution often being taken is for the patient to wear an ID card in the neck or placed in the pocket. This contains the name, address and contact person of who should be called when this happens.

The sixth stage of Alzheimer's is when the person also begins to have mood swings. The patient may be jolly to talking to other people when suddenly everything changes and the attitude is now hostile to whoever is there.

The worse part about the disorder during this stage is that the person will act like a baby. Tantrums may be thrown but the worst part is seeing the patient defecate on his or herself. The caretaker will have to clean up the mess as though the person was an infant and are advised to use adult diapers, which is more convenient when cleaning up the mess.

The seventh stage of Alzheimer's is not that bad anymore. This is because the body's systems will slowly shut down. The patient won't speak or do anything and will usually just stare into space.

It is like the person gave up the will to live. The body may be there but the mind or the soul has gone off to another place.

Anyone who is diagnosed with Alzheimer's will have less than 10 years left to live. Doctors only catch on in the third and fourth stages since the symptoms of short-term memory loss are hardly noticeable and often attributed to aging.

What can people do for those who have Alzheimer's? Unfortunately, there is not that much anyone can do because there is no cure yet for this disorder. There are drugs available that can only slow down the process before it gets worse but those who care are just delaying the inevitable.

Research shows that there are more than four million people in the country that are suffering from this disease. The figure will go higher as the baby boom generation also reaches the same age.

As long as there are drugs that can delay the process, doctors may be able to buy a little more time so that the person may live to see the day that a cure has been made.

Alzheimer's Disease and Its Symptoms

Alzheimer's disease, also known as the most common form of dementia, is named after the German neurologist Dr. Alois Alzheimer who first identified the disease in 1907. The main concern with Alzheimer's disease is that it allows the rapid degeneration of healthy brain tissue associated with cognitive abilities such as judgment, comprehension and memory.

The root cause of this phenomenon in Alzheimer's disease remains unclear and is still under study. This degeneration of the brain tissues causes a steady decline in memory as well as a steady loss of essential mental abilities responsible for thought, memory, and language. More than four million of the older population in the US is known to be stricken with Alzheimer's disease. The number of people suffering from this debilitating condition is expected to triple within the next 20 years.

The most common symptoms of Alzheimer's are loss of memory, the decline of intellectual functions and sudden changes in personality. At the first stages of the disease, symptoms exhibited are patients becoming easily tired, upset and anxious.

With Alzheimer's disease the changes that happen may be gradual over time and not so sudden. But as the disease progresses, so does the Alzheimer's symptoms as they accelerate and become more serious and noticeable enough for the people involved to seek help. The usual course of the disease can take anything from five to ten years, from how the Alzheimer's symptoms develop from simple forgetfulness to showing up as severe dementia.

On the part of the patient, the initial Alzheimer's symptom that can be very frightening is the realization that something is happening to their memory. Although simple forgetfulness is not the only Alzheimer's symptom to look for, but it reaches the degree as even forgetting the names of people that the patient sees often, then the condition is a possible Alzheimer's symptom. The Alzheimer's symptom starts off with slight memory loss and confusion. It then ultimately leads to severe and irreversible mental impairment if left to develop without any form of initial treatment.

The Alzheimer's symptom will further lead to degeneration of a person's ability to remember, reason, learn and even imagine. The Alzheimer's symptom of forgetfulness can include the names of family members being forgotten as well as familiar everyday objects such as a comb and mirror.

Another possible symptom of the disease includes difficulty experienced with abstract thinking. This symptom initially begins with typically mundane everyday things like not balancing a check book and may further develop into not understanding and recognizing numbers.

Difficulty finding the right word can also be an Alzheimer's symptom that challenges the patient with finding the correct words for expression. It will eventually lead to a diminished ability to follow conversations and further progress to affect one's reading and writing skills. Those with Alzheimer's may have trouble finding the right words to identify objects, express thoughts or take part in conversations. Over time, the ability to read and write also declines.

Disorientation with time and dates is also an evident symptom of Alzheimer's; even further deteriorating to the degree as to frequently losing themselves in even very familiar surroundings.

Loss of judgment is an Alzheimer's symptom that prevents the patient from solving everyday problems and doing simple tasks like cooking on the stove. This Alzheimer's symptom in its extreme form will lead to difficulty with anything that requires planning, decision-making and judgment.

Personality change is an Alzheimer's symptom that presents itself as the gradual development of mood swings, distrust, stubbornness and eventual withdrawal from the patient's usual social circle. Depression is also a coexistent Alzheimer's symptom alongside with growing restlessness. In its severe form, the Alzheimer's symptom further develops into anxiety, aggressiveness and inappropriate behavior.

Once-routine activities that require sequential steps, such as planning and cooking a meal or playing a favourite game, become a struggle as the disease progresses. Eventually, people with advanced Alzheimer's may forget how to perform basic tasks such as dressing and bathing.

Cause of Alzheimer's Disease

Alzheimer's disease is a form of a mental disorder that is also known as "dementia", a brain disorder that affects and seriously impedes the brain's ability to process rational or normal thought. This usually results in limiting the amount of daily activities that require the use of cognitive abilities of its sufferers. Alzheimer's is a debilitating disease because it affects the part of the brain that is responsible for thought, memory, and language.

Alzheimer's is especially one of the most disabling diseases that can affect the older population. What makes Alzheimer's disease a very serious affliction is that it is a progressive disorder that can slowly kill the irreplaceable nerve cells in the brain. Although Alzheimer's is detected more often among patients over 60 years old, there are some individuals as young as 50 years of age who can show signs of Alzheimer's.

Alzheimer's disease holds no boundaries. It can equally affect people of different cultures and is found to afflict both males and females in equal proportions. Not one particular test is known to be used for diagnosing Alzheimer's. A variety of methods and tests are being used to diagnose 90 percent of Alzheimer's cases. A 100 percent accuracy in diagnosing the disease can only be achieved upon autopsy to check for plaques and tangles in the sufferer's brain.

The root cause of Alzheimer's disease is not yet quite well understood despite the many years of research on the debilitating condition. Alzheimer's is a complex disease that can be caused by a number of different influences.

The main cause of Alzheimer's disease that researchers today have found out is damaged brain cells that die for unknown reasons. The cause of Alzheimer's disease, which was first isolated by the German neurologist Dr. Alois Alzheimer, is the abnormal clumping together of brain cells. These clumps, also known as plaques, and knots or tangles which disrupt normal brain functioning, are considered as the main definitive characteristics of Alzheimer's disease.

Alzheimer's Disease and Its Cause

Genetics are also being studied as a possible cause of Alzheimer's disease. Another possible cause of the disease is seen to be a slow developing viral infection that results in brain inflammation. Although the actual cause of Alzheimer's disease may not yet be known and still in the discovery stages, there are a number of risk factors that is known to increase the likelihood of Alzheimer development.

Age is known as a risk cause of Alzheimer's disease. As a person ages, the likelihood that he or she will develop Alzheimer's also increases. The average age of diagnosis for Alzheimer's is about 80 years old. Gender is also seen as involved in the development of Alzheimer's disease, but studies for this may still be inconclusive. The reason as to why the risk is seen to be greater in women is that they tend to live longer than the men.

Hereditary tendency is being looked into as another risk cause of Alzheimer's disease. The presence of some defective genes and genetic mutations within the same bloodlines has also been seen to increase the development of Alzheimer's disease.

Another possible cause of Alzheimer's disease that is being looked into is the malfunction of the immune system and protein imbalances that occur in the brain. Certain environmental factors such as the presence of aluminum in the home or workplace are also being put under investigation as a possible cause of Alzheimer's disease.

Alzheimer's Testing

Alzheimer's is a disease that robs millions of people each year of their memories, their personalities, and the ability to complete daily activities. The disease can greatly affect the quality of life of every sufferer as well as those people around him, most especially immediate family members.

For a long time, most people believe that there is nothing that could be done to prevent this awful disease. People came to accept it as a result of deteriorating of mental abilities due to age. It was considered as simply something that people had to cope up with when approaching their golden years of life. But doctors today have discovered and now consider Alzheimer's as a disease that can be treated up to a certain extent.

The hallmark sign associated with Alzheimer's disease is the gradual loss of memory especially in people of 65 years and older. Although forgetfulness is a sign of the said disease, it should also be noted that there are other signs that may also indicate the onset of this ailment. Before coming up with your own conclusions, it is best to know more about Alzheimer's through its exhibited signs, how it can be diagnosed and how it will eventually affects the sufferer.

Diagnosis of Alzheimer's disease can be done through a series of tests. The patient exhibiting some signs of the disease must undergo a variety of laboratory tests, such as physical and mental assessments. As of late, there is no known single test available that will effectively diagnose Alzheimer's in patients.

But with recent developments and advances in the medical field, doctors have been able to devise a set of Alzheimer's disease testing tools that can help in effectively detect symptoms of the disease in its earlier stages.

As of yet, there is no single definitive test that is able to determine if one has Alzheimer's disease. But it is really a battery of testing that is available that makes it possible for physicians to diagnose Alzheimer's with about 90 percent accuracy. Such battery of tests can take anywhere from one day to several weeks in order to ensure accuracy and the proper diagnosis.

Among the various tests available there is one set of tests that has recently been developed that will further help make diagnosing Alzheimer's disease easier. A professor of psychology at Williams College in Williamstown, Massachusetts, has developed a new tool for testing called the Seven Minute Screen that can test people for the early signs of Alzheimer's disease as well as other forms of dementia.

The said test, developed by Paul Solomon, is actually a set of four tests that can be administered to patients in just less than ten minutes, can also be completed on average of just seven minutes and forty three seconds. What makes the said test even more convenient is that it can be administered by any medical professional with just over an hour of basic training.

The short time that it takes for completing the whole test is an attractive option for doctors who may not have the luxury of time when they are diagnosing patients with Alzheimer's.

This type of test is just a part of a much larger effort by medical researchers to develop better ways of detecting Alzheimer's early. A likely option that some researchers are trying to look into is the use of brain scanning technology such as magnetic resonance imaging or MRI to identify even the smallest damage to the brain before any impairment in cognitive ability ever show up in people likely to develop Alzheimer's. Other possible approaches being studied involve looking for gene abnormalities in patients that have been linked to Alzheimer's disease.

Your doctor may recommend a more extensive assessment of your thinking and memory. Longer forms of neuropsychological testing, which can take several hours to complete, may provide additional details about your mental function compared with others' of a similar age and education level. This type of testing may be especially helpful if your doctor thinks you may have a very early stage of Alzheimer's disease or another dementia. These tests may also help identify patterns of change associated with different types of dementia.

Researchers are working with doctors to develop new diagnostic tools to help clinch the diagnosis of Alzheimer's. Another important goal is to detect the disease before it causes the symptoms targeted by current diagnostic techniques — at the stage when Alzheimer's may be most treatable as new drugs are discovered. New tools under investigation include: Additional approaches to brain imaging, Measuring levels of key proteins or protein patterns in blood or spinal fluid and More-sensitive mental status tests.

Living with Alzheimer's Disease

When someone is diagnosed with Alzheimer's disease, those around should not think that it is the end of the world. The best thing to do is help the one who is suffering from it until the person dies.

There are drugs in the market that can help ease the pain but not reverse the process or stop the disease from spreading. The only thing it can do is slow down the process that could buy enough time until a cure has been found.

Family members should give this or hire a caregiver to do that when no one is able to take care of the person.

In time, the sufferer may not even recall the name of the children. One way to help the one living with Alzheimer's is through the use of visual aids. The name and the picture of the person can be shown in a card and someone can conduct memory exercises on the individual.

It will also be a good idea to talk as often as possible with the patient. The person should be within the line of sight of the individual and must say each word slowly in order to understand each word being said.

The best place to treat someone with Alzheimer's is in the home. The people who are there should make sure that there is order in the house and it is quiet at all times because noise will just aggravate the patient.

Living with someone who has Alzheimer's can be compared to taking care of a toddler. This is because the person will touch anything in sight and might even get hurt in the process. The best thing to do is to take make sure there is no clutter in the house and items that are deemed unsafe are hidden from view.

Alzheimer sufferers are known to wander off. The person can lock the doors but should the patient manage to get out, it is best to have either a bracelet or a pocket card inserted in the clothing. This must have the name, address of the patient as well as the contact number where someone can be reached to pick up the wanderer.

Studies show that those who are suffering from Alzheimer's disease really get worked up in the evening. This can be prevented by coming up with evening rituals such as washing the dishes, watching television or walking around for a while to make the patient calm and sleep tight.

Those who are suffering from Alzheimer's aside from the medicine prescribed by the doctor also need exercise. It doesn't have to be anything extraneous but just enough to keep the strength up. An early morning walk or lifting small weights are just a few examples to promote a certain level of fitness for the patient.

It is not easy living with someone who has Alzheimer's disease because the task of taking care of someone is both tiring and frustrating. People have to understand that no one wanted this to happen but the reality is that the problem is there.

It is a good thing there are support groups out there that can help family members and patients cope with this disease. The people can also live closer because it won't be long before the inevitable will happen and this person will go off to a better place.

Treatment and Care for Alzheimer's Patients

Many breakthroughs and important discoveries have been found throughout the years of research and testing regarding the cure and treatment of Alzheimer's disease. Despite that though, there continues to be no known cure or prevention for Alzheimer's. Furthermore, once the disease has started, there can be no repairing or slowing down the damage of abnormal deposits of proteins in the brain.

People with Alzheimer's have abnormal deposits of protein in their brains. This brain protein coats the brain and interacts with the neurons, neurotransmitters and nerves, causing damage and massive atrophy. Eventually, the brain will continue to shrink and the otherwise wrinkled surface will start to smoothen out. This is basically what causes the degeneration in the mind and in the person's body.

There however are some drugs and treatments that seem to relieve symptomatic conditions slightly in some cases. These drugs and Alzheimer's treatments are especially important during the onset and early stages of the illness when the sufferer can still be aware of what he or she is going through.

For instance, a person with Alzheimer's at the early stages may suffer from depression or restlessness and certain drugs and Alzheimer's treatments can be administered to help with this somewhat. Also, there have been some cases where memory loss at the beginning of dementia can still be improved somehow. Other possible symptoms that can be momentarily alleviated are sleep disorders and hallucinations.

Beyond these, the proper Alzheimer's treatment of caregivers for patients is a highly specialized skill and needs to be administered by a professional. This will mean that the patient will eventually have to be entrusted in institutionalized care for the proper Alzheimer's treatment needed.

Of course, loved ones of the Alzheimer's patient will want to administer care personally but the care and Alzheimer's treatment needed by the patient will be full time and specialized so it is best for a professional caregiver to ensure dignity is maintained throughout the course of the person's disease.

Despite the present lack of Alzheimer's treatment and cure, hope should never be abandoned. After all the technological advancements that have been made in the field of science and medicine, it probably won't be long before the proper Alzheimer's treatment and cure will be discovered.

If not the cure or Alzheimer's treatment, then perhaps the methods of prevention against Alzheimer's will be found to help other individuals not fall into this predicament. Perhaps in the near future, there will be vaccines for Alzheimer's disease much like we all have vaccines against diseases like small pox and the like. All those diseases in the past posed a challenge to humanity then just like Alzheimer's does now.

In the meantime, if you or someone you know and care about suffers from Alzheimer's, it is best to consult a professional for possible options for instance for eventual institutional care, or for support groups or counseling advice that can be given to the patient and to his or her friends and relatives.

There may be some misconceptions and even some difficulty in accepting the situation of this disease whether it is on the side of the patient or from the people around him or her. For instances such as these, the right counseling and guidance is needed as part of the proper Alzheimer's treatment.

Drugs to Fight Alzheimer's

Although there is no known cure yet for Alzheimer's disease, there are already a number of drugs available worldwide that can help slow down a patient's cognitive deterioration. The main aim of these Alzheimer's medications is to try and improve cognitive ability or the person's capability to think, perceive, judge and recognize.

There are currently five drugs approved by the Food and Drug Administration (FDA) that can be used to treat Alzheimer's. There is ongoing research done all the time to test the effectiveness of such medications since they do not serve as a cure-all for the disease.

These medications may not have the same effects on all patients that are suffering from Alzheimer's. But such prescription drugs can have significant effects on some of the patients with Alzheimer's disease and should be given consideration as a possible treatment.

The 5 FDA Approved Medications are:

Aricept

Cognex

Exelon

Razadyne

Namenda

The first four drugs listed above belong to a group of drugs known as Cholinesterase Inhibitors. They work by trying to delay the breakdown of a substance known as acetylcholine in the brain which helps in bridging communication between nerve cells and has an important role in a person's memory.

Nameda on the other hand acts on another neurotransmitter called glutamate and shields the brain from then said substance which contributes to the death of brain cells in people with Alzheimer's disease. This drug is more effective in treating moderate to severe forms of Alzheimer's disease, improving the day to day life of the person with Alzheimer's disease.

The most common side effects associated with the drug Nameda include dizziness, confusion, constipation, headache and skin rashes. Some patients may experience less common side effects such as tiredness, back pain, high blood pressure, insomnia, hallucinations, vomiting and occasional shortness of breath.

The drugs Aricept, Exelon and Razadyne are seen to be most effective in treating the early stages of Alzheimer's disease. This group of prescription drugs has been shown to have some modest effect in slowing down the degeneration of a patient's cognitive abilities.

These drugs can also help in trying to reduce certain behavioral problems usually exhibited by people suffering from Alzheimer's. When these drugs are administered effectively on an Alzheimer's patient, they can significantly improve one's quality of life and more able to cope up with the disease.

Alzheimer's patients taking these medications may experience some side effects which may not be the same for all patients. Common side effects observed in patients using the drug Aricept include nausea, vomiting, excessive tiredness, sleeping troubles and muscle cramps.

Less frequent observed side effects of the drug are headaches and dizziness with rare cases of patients suffering from anorexia, gastric or duodenal ulcers, gastro-intestinal hemorrhage, bladder overflow obstruction, liver damage, convulsions, heart problems and psychiatric disturbances while using Aricept as medication.

The usual side effects seen in using Exelon as treatment for Alzheimer's are nausea, vomiting, weight loss, stomach upset and fatigue. Less usual side effects observed with the use of the said drug are abdominal pain, sweating, diarrhea, headaches, tremor, and psychiatric disturbances such as anxiety or depression with rare cases of patients experiencing gastro-intestinal bleeding.

The drug Cognex is used less frequently for Alzheimer's treatment as it can cause serious liver damage to most patients. Other side effects of the drug include nausea and vomiting. Some patients may also experience some abdominal pain, sore muscles, headache, dizziness, rapid breathing, increased urination, insomnia, runny nose or mouth, swelling in legs and feet when taking Cognex. Some of the most severe side effects associated with using Cornex are liver damage, heart problems and seizures.

The common side effects often reported with the use of Razadyne are nausea, vomiting, appetite loss and weight loss. Less common are fatigue, dizziness, tremor, headaches, abdominal pain, urinary tract infection, blood in urine, runny nose. There are no serious side effects with this drug.

Drugs as a Treatment for Alzheimer's

As more and more individuals are diagnosed with the debilitating Alzheimer's disease, more and more information are coming up as scientists and researchers continue to find out more about this enigmatic type of dementia. Despite this however, a lot of questions remain unanswered. These unanswered questions are hampering experts from finding out the cause of the disease as well as the cure.

What is known for a fact is that individuals begin to become susceptible to the disease at the age of 65 and above. It is also known that Alzheimer's disease attack the brain and causes an abnormality there, which in turn causes the loss of normal functions in the body.

When a person has Alzheimer's, he or she will have an abnormal deposit of brain protein that destroys the brain's neurons, nerves and neurotransmitters. An autopsy of the brain of the person who suffered from Alzheimer's will show a decrease of brain size and a smoother surface.

If experts can absolutely conclude on the causes of Alzheimer's then perhaps an Alzheimer's drug as a vaccine can be administered to individuals to be able to inhibit the ailment from happening. The statistics on Alzheimer's cases are starting to raise much concern because care for individuals with this disease can rake up a lot of money that may in turn put a dent on a country's health care system funds because of the alarming number of cases of individuals with Alzheimer's.

Intensive care and costs are entailed for individuals who suffer from this because although at the onset and mild stage of the disease, only a slight short term memory loss is perceived, eventually the sufferer will lose more and more cognitive abilities. The person will begin to forget things more and more and will even begin to lose recognition of people and things that are a close part of his or life. There will also be marked instances of uncontrollable changes in behavior.

As the disease advances, the Alzheimer's sufferer will begin to lose more and more motor skills and the ability to function independently from another. They will then have to be cared for by qualified caregivers who will have to take care of getting them fed and mobile when needed.

Aside from this though, the most imperative need for concrete answers in terms of Alzheimer's drug treatments lies in the fact that this disease is irreversible and inexorably progresses into death. At present, Alzheimer's disease has no known cure and Alzheimer's drug treatments give only slight symptomatic relief for some patients but in no way can it buy an individual more time.

This claim has been debated however by pharmaceutical companies. For more information about Alzheimer's drug treatments: what has been observed to work and what hasn't; check out literature on The American Association for Geriatric Psychiatry's official statement.

There is no reason to lose hope however because involved sectors are doing all they can to be able to conquer this disease. As more and more breakthroughs on the subject arise, there is no doubt that perhaps in the near future, an Alzheimer's drug will be found successful in treating and curing this disease. In the meantime, friends, loved ones and caregivers of individuals with Alzheimer's need to stay abreast of the latest news and breakthroughs in the field of Alzheimer's research.

The latest (2011) guidance from the National Institute for Health and Clinical Excellence (NICE) recommends that donepezil, rivastigmine and galantamine are available as part of NHS care for people with mild-to-moderate Alzheimer's disease. There are also now several studies – including work supported by Alzheimer's Society – which suggest that cholinesterase inhibitors may also help people with more severe Alzheimer's disease. However, these drugs are not licensed in the UK for the treatment of severe Alzheimer's disease.

Between 40 and 70 per cent of people with Alzheimer's disease benefit from cholinesterase inhibitor treatment, but it is not effective for everyone and may improve symptoms only temporarily, between six and 12 months in most cases. According to an Alzheimer's Society survey of 4,000 people, those using these treatments often experience improvements in motivation, anxiety levels and confidence, in addition to daily living, memory and thinking.

It is not clear whether the cholinesterase inhibitors bring benefits for behavioural symptoms such as agitation or aggression. Trials have given mixed results here. Research does suggest that these drugs (and memantine) bring some relief from the carer's perspective.

Memantine is licensed for the treatment of moderate-to-severe Alzheimer's disease. It can temporarily slow down the progression of symptoms, including everyday function, in people in the middle and later stages of the disease.

Preventing Alzheimer's Disease

When one reaches the later years of one's life, systems will slow down and bones will weaken. This is the time when you will not be able to do the things that you used to do before or if you were still able to do it, you would not be able to do it with the same speed and strength as you used to before.

That is the sad fact about aging. Things will slow down and eventually, little by little, disappear.

But that is not always the case. For some people, the aging process can speed up especially in the area of the brain.

This is what scientists call Alzheimer's.

It is a degenerative and progressive disease that targets the brain, particularly the areas that deal with learning and memory. Although it often affects people over the age of 80, there are some who are diagnosed with the problem as early as their 40s and 50s. There are also rare cases when Alzheimer's attacks at late 20s.

Alzheimer's Disease is characterized by a progressive memory loss and inability to focus attention on one thing. People with this disease will forget their names, their addresses and will cease to recognize their husbands, children and people who are close to them.

When it is on its later stages, language problems may also happen because of the inability of the person to recall words that are appropriate for what they are going to say. The disease may also result to behavioral changes because of progressive memory loss. There are some patients who don't remember how to go about their normal functions such as eating, sleeping or brushing their teeth. Some may even forget how to breathe.

This is the reason why most old people dread this disease. It can really be debilitating, robbing you of your life and often times your loved one.

Although nothing has been proven yet, some studies show that doing mental tasks can actually slow down the progression of the disease. For instance, patients who love to answer puzzles and play mental games like chess are slower in their progression compared to other patients with the same degree and case of Alzheimer. Because of this, some scientists believe that Alzheimer's can be prevented through the use of the mental process.

Below are some ways to prevent Alzheimer's from settling in.

Learn Something New

Old age is not a reason to stop learning new things. You can learn a variety of things, dancing, cooking, singing, a new language, crafts, the arts. There are so many things to choose from. Don the things that you have not done before, things that you never thought you'll be doing. Your age should not be hindrance to the things that you want to do.

In addition to enriching your life, learning something new affords a fresh challenge for your brains. This way, your mental processes will be used once again. This keeps the brain cells in shape and sharp.

Play Mind Games

This is not to say that you should be scheming and plotting, stirring the boat for the members of your family. Mind games here refer to the tamer kind, crossword puzzles, sudoku. These are ways to sharpen those mental skills and memory. This also allows you to practice or be familiar with words and things once again, lessening the chance of you forgetting them.

Who Are You? Alzheimer's Symptoms

From the German psychiatrist who first diagnosed the disease, Alzheimer's is a fatal disease that has both no known cause and cure. There are treatments that help prevent the disease to develop into its complete form. Plus medications already exists which could assist patients to manage their agitation, depression, hallucinations or delusions which could manifest during the later stages of the disease.

There are a number of symptoms which help diagnose the disease. The most prominent of which is memory loss. What seems to be a simple lapse in memory could be the start of Alzheimer's disease. Loss of memory in Alzheimer's is manifested from the more than unusual fluctuating forgetfulness to short-term memory loss.

Later, the patient will start to forget familiar things and well-known skills. They will start to forget names, objects, and persons even those that are close to them. Alzheimer's memory loss is often accompanied by aphasia, disorientation and disinhibition. Aside from forgetfulness and amnesia, some refer to Alzheimer's related memory loss as memory decay, memory decline, or memory impairment (Loring, 1999).

One, however, should not conclude that all memory loss is caused by Alzheimer's disease. There are two basic causes of memory loss, namely normal or age related memory loss and the abnormal type. It is normal that middle age and older people begin to forget a number of things. Their ability to remember is often times measured on a standardized scale.

If their memory scores fall within the designated cut-off, their memory loss is due to normal and age-related causes. Meanwhile, if they fail to pass the scores it means that their memory loss is caused by not mere age-related reasons but by abnormal, or age-inappropriate, memory disease or impairment instead. One, therefore, needs to let professional medical workers to isolate and determine if he/she got Alzheimer's disease.

Aside from the early symptom of memory loss, Alzheimer's disease at the early stage could also change the patient's behavior. And as the disease develops, the patient will lose more and more control over body functions such as affecting the way the person thinks and respond. With the effects on the brain's cognitive functions, the patient will have trouble talking, will find skilled movements troublesome to do and hard to accomplish, and will start slowing down in terms of movements.

The patient will become indecisive and will start having trouble in decision-making processes and planning stages of human activities. These losses of memory and cognitive functions are related to the frontal and temporal lobes of the brain. The two lobes are becoming disconnected from the limbic system due to the disease.

Also, part of the symptoms of Alzheimer's is mood swings and outbursts of violence or excessive passivity. The later stages will be more horrible. People with Alzheimer's will later on start to loose bowel movement as well as muscle control and mobility. Alzheimer's usually develops and become fatal within approximately 7–10 years.

Since Dr. Alzheimer diagnosed the disease in 1901, there have been a lot of medical discoveries and tons of results from research studies and medical investigations that were found to be beneficial in preventing or delaying Alzheimer's disease.

Studies found out that exercise helps lessen the risk of contracting the disease. Scientists have found significant findings which indicate that having high blood pressure, high cholesterol, and low levels of the vitamin folate can increase one's risk of acquiring Alzheimer's disease.

More About Alzheimer's Disease

People tend to forget certain things because of work and other priorities. This is not uncommon because this does happen to everybody. However, when an individual tends to forget even the simplest things, there is already something definitely wrong. There is a chance that one has Alzheimer's disease.

Alzheimer's disease is a disorder in the brain. In time, the patient will gradually lose both the intellectual and social abilities making it difficult to do anything and even interact with others.

This disease commonly afflicts people above 65 years of age. There are currently 4.5 million Americans that are suffering from this disease. It is projected that this number will increase, as the more population will reach the retirement age.

There is no known cure yet for Alzheimer's disease. The only thing medical science can do for now is simply delay the inevitable for those who have just been diagnosed with the disease.

Is Alzheimer's disease the same as dementia? The answer is no. This is because dementia is a symptom, which is caused by a disorder such as Alzheimer's disease.

There are many symptoms for this disease. It may begin with the person simply forgetting certain things. It is hard to tell at this point but when it gets worse such as not knowing how to get to the office or get home, then there is definitely a problem.

Some patients are known to forget how to do some simple mathematical computations or even find the right words when writing a letter. There are those who are also disoriented and find it difficult to do certain tasks and make simple decisions.

The worse of these symptoms is perhaps experiencing personality changes even in the presence of family members and close friends. There are times the person is happy and then this will just change for no reason at all.

A neurological scan is the best way to check if the patient has Alzheimer's disease. If it is confirmed, the individual has this problem, the best way to treat it is through the use of medical prescribed drugs.

There are two namely memantine and cholinesterase inhibitors. Studies have shown these can slow down the process as scientists are still conducting research to finally find a cure for this disease.

Patients who are diagnosed with the disorder will probably live more for 8 more years. This will really depend on how strong the person is because some have lived for 3 while others have fought with it for more than 10 years.

How can family members help a loved one with this disease? The siblings can take turns watching over the patient. If this is not possible, this is the time that a caregiver must be hired to check on the patient. This specialist will usually stay in the home and make sure the person is safe.

Physical and mental exercises must be administered to keep the patient's strength up and even help depression, which is another symptom commonly, associated with Alzheimer's disease.

Whenever the people visit, it is best for each person to stay in the line of sight of the patient. It is best to speak slowly and even hold on to the individual, which is known to make the sufferer remember who he or she is talking to.

Alzheimer's and Dementia

Alzheimer's and dementia are strongly linked because Alzheimer's disease is the most common type of dementia. Dementia is the constant evolution of the atrophy of the brain's cognitive functions. In the case of Alzheimer's, abnormal protein build up happen in the brain which interferes with its normal functions through interactions with the brain nerves and neurotransmitters that cause these elements to wither and die.

Alzheimer's and dementia are attributed with progressive memory loss and other functions that are attributed to brain deterioration. Natural brain atrophy and cognitive function loss is a normal experience by humans as we age. However, Alzheimer's type of dementia is way beyond that of what is considered the norm.

Alzheimer's type dementia is extremely debilitating and the disease can run its course from as fast as 5 years but some cases stretch on to 20 years. The disruption of Alzheimer's type dementia can be very confusing and difficult. What's really hard to accept is that as of the moment, there are no known cures or successful treatments available for Alzheimer's patients.

Of all the types of dementia, only a very tiny percentage is reversible and Alzheimer's is not one of them. Once it attacks, there can be no slowing or stopping down. All one can do is be prepared for the onslaught. In this case, it is also important the patient's friends and loved one understand and know all about Alzheimer's and dementia so that they too can be allowed to cope with this situation.

If you suffer from the very early stages of Alzheimer's type dementia, it can be very difficult for you to accept what is happening to you while you are aware of your situation. Often times, patients can create very difficult situations for themselves as well as for the people around them. For instance, people with Alzheimer's type dementia can have the same conversation with the same person over and over again without realizing it.

Perhaps a person with Alzheimer's type dementia can forget that they have just previously called a loved one to tell them something only to put the phone down and call right back to talk about the exact same thing. Situations like these can cause difficulties; that is why it is important for people with Alzheimer's type dementia to have the proper care.

Loss of correct judgment will inadvertently follow as the Alzheimer's type dementia progresses so it might be prudent for patients to be supervised all the time. Eventually, patients will have to depend exclusively on specialized care for all their needs. This makes it important for patients and their loved ones to choose the right facility for this process.

It is important that people with Alzheimer's type dementia be treated with respect and dignity all throughout the duration of the disease. While the patient has not lost all ability to make judgments and remember important things, they should be consulted in terms of what facilities or type of professional care they think they would benefit from.

As a loved one of someone who has Alzheimer's type dementia, it can be very hard and painful to witness the progressing of the disease. This may cause some negative emotions and a lot of grief that may be unwittingly projected at the patient.

However, at the onset of the disease, when the patient is still conscious and aware, they can go through an even more painful process of accepting their disease.

Alzheimer's Care Facility

More than 4 million Americans are suffering from Alzheimer's disease. Statistics show that the number of sufferers will continue to increase as more people will reach the retirement age.

People who are diagnosed with the disorder do not have to be confined in the hospital. The best Alzheimer's care facility does not cost much because the patient can be treated in the comforts of one's home.

What are the changes that need to be done to the home? The good news is, none. Those who are taking care of the patient should just be sure it is clean, clutter and noise free at all times.

If the family members are busy with other things, an ad can be placed in the paper or someone can call the agency to have a caregiver look after the sufferer. These specialists are trained to give aid to the patient.

What activities are done in the care facility? For starters, memory exercises will be done so the patient can still remember the names of the family members. A basic one will be through the use of flash cards that have the name and photo of the person.

Most of the time, the caretaker will be beside the patient. Instead of doing nothing, it wouldn't hurt to strike up a conversation. It does not have to be anything serious but just enough to keep the person active because an inactive mind may lead to depression.

The individual should always make eye-to-eye contact when talking to the patient at the same time speaking slowly and clearly for the other person to understand.

Alzheimer sufferers tend to wander off. The patient could walk to the end of the street or even walk farther without the caretaker even knowing and that is worse. A failsafe system must be put in place such as making sure the doors and windows are locked at all times.

Should the patient manage to get out, the second fail-safe will be to attach a bracelet or a card. This will make it easy for someone to return the person home or be informed where the sufferer can be picked up.

The Alzheimer's care facility is open 24/7 with most of the concentration spent at night. This is because the symptoms are more active during this time so the best way to calm the patient down is through a little exercise.

The patient can help do the dishes or work on the laundry. A cup of warm milk or tea can be given. If this doesn't work, perhaps going for a little stroll together outside for a little exercise may make the sufferer sleepy and go off to bed.

Some states have nursing homes and reputable home care facilities to treat the patient. There are numbers in the directory as well as in the Internet that people can inquire.

The individual should not be surprised should the place not accept just anyone who can no longer take on the burden of taking care of the loved one because of the limited space and the stage of the disease.

The person can choose to pay a huge sum or spend the remaining days with the loved one close to home to at least have a few good memories until the patient will finally go off to a better place.

Finding Caregivers

One of the most dreaded diseases in old age is Alzheimer's disease. Although unlike cancer and heart problem, this is actually not fatal. In fact, people with Alzheimer's can live for a long time with proper care. That is actually the problem most of the time.

With Alzheimer's disease, the patient needs to be taken care of all the time. This is because the memory loss will often render the patient incapable of thinking and reasoning. Some will even forget how to do the simplest of tasks, like brushing their teeth and even eating with a spoon and fork.

Alzheimer's is a progressive and degenerative disease that affects the brain. The problem often leads to massive memory loss not only in terms of one's memories but also one's learning. Patients will forget everything that they have learned even routinely tasks that they have learned when they were just tots. Some people will also find it hard to learn new things and may even lose their language abilities. They will have difficulties in their speech and in their writing.

Because of this, caring for a patient with Alzheimer's disease can be extremely difficult. It is actually like caring for a newborn babe but while a baby will slowly learn to function independently, patients with Alzheimer's will lose what they have learned and will slowly become more and more dependent with their caregivers. Thus, it is important to find a caregiver that is both professionally-capable and caring as they will determine the progress that the patient will have as well as their overall condition and behavior.

Here are some tips in finding a good caregiver for an Alzheimer's patient.

Choose a Professional

It is good to look for a person that is already well experienced in caring for people with Alzheimer's. Not only will their experience come in handy when it comes to dealing with the patient's medicines and medical routines, they will also be more patient because of prior knowledge.

One problem though in hiring these kinds of people is the money that you will shell out for their salaries. Private Nurses and caregivers are expensive enough as it is without adding the burden of a specialization. If you just cannot afford to hire someone with enough experience, try one who has worked with old people and then give him or her materials that will make them familiar with the basics of the disease.

Choose Someone You Know

Nothing beats hiring someone that you already know or someone that you have already seen working. Patients with Alzheimer's will have a lot of quirks and behavior that can be extremely irritating and difficult to deal with. Thus, it is important that you choose someone that you know will have a lot of patience and care.

Of course, if a member of the family can spare the time for the patient, it is good. If not, you can ask for recommendations from people that you know. Chances are they know someone who can take care of a patient with Alzheimer's.

Choose Someone Strong

Although this is actually not a major issue, it is also important that you choose someone who can deal with the patient and the often back breaking tasks. Remember that because the patient is full- dependent on the person, they will sometimes need to carry them or guide them when walking.

Keeping People with Alzheimer's Busy

Alzheimer's disease is considered the 7th leading cause of death in the United States in 2004. The death toll continues to rise every year. The disease is the third most costly in the U.S. Heart disease and cancer are the first and second most costly respectively. It is recorded that there 24 million people with dementia worldwide, the figure will more than double by 2040.

Alzheimer's is a progressive disease that is irreversible with no known cause or cure. The disease affects two major types of abilities. Alzheimer's affects the very simple everyday activities such as dressing, eating, bathing, dressing, using the toilet, and even walking. One needs to be assisted in order to accomplish such tasks.

The other ability affected by the disease are the performance of more complex tasks like managing finances, driving a car, preparing and cooking meals and working in a job. It is normal for people with the disease to experience problems with complex tasks first which later on move to the more simple everyday jobs as the disease progresses.

Treatment is vital for people with Alzheimer's disease. Treating a patient requires the conglomeration of the expertise of a family doctor and various medical specialists like psychiatrists or neurologists, psychologists, therapists, nurses, social workers, and counselors; because the disease affects not only the patient but the whole family as well.

It is very important that family members work closely with the doctors in administering the treatment. The family should be informed of activities that are dangerous for people with Alzheimer's disease. Some of these activities include driving or cooking.

Treating dementia related symptoms of Alzheimer's vary. But such treatments can only be effective if the dementia is caused by factors like medications, alcohol, delirium, tumors, depression, head injury and infections. There are, however, some treatments that are being used to "cure" the well-being of a person afflicted with the disease.

Activities like playing music, personal interactions, playing videotapes of family members, walking and light exercise and pet therapy have been found to be successful in helping people develop friendship, mutual support and spiritual connectedness with the people around them.

However, one should remember that such activities can be beneficial to one but could be detrimental to another patient. The best activity for a person with Alzheimer's varies. Former hobbies or points of interest of a person could also be used to help people with the disease and their families to cope.

One could assist the person to engage in activities like supervised gardening, singing, cooking, painting and drawing as long as routine is established. It is very important to engage in these activities on a regular basis for this could help the person establish a sense of stability.

Some therapies combine various activities and have proved to be fairly successful and garnered some favorable results. Such programs combine music, exercise, crafts and relaxation which obtained the best results.

Some even add various structured sessions like meditations, sensory awareness and guided imagery in their attempts to calm and pacify the already unstable behaviors of patients with Alzheimer's.

Aside from daily physical exercise and social activities, some of the things that you also need to consider in treating a patient are proper nutrition and health maintenance; daily activities that will give the feelings of accomplishment for the individual; keeping the patient out of harm's way; and knowing the physical and emotional limitations of the patient, the care giver team and the family.

Activities for People with Alzheimer

Alzheimer's is one disease that people dread to be diagnosed with. Who can blame them?

It is one of the most debilitating diseases known to man and it affects not only one area or one system but all. Of course, since it is a progressive disease, effects on the various systems of the body does not happen at one time.

As the disease progress, the effects become wide-range.

Alzheimer's disease is perhaps the best-known disease under Dementia, a disorder that affects the mental processes. It is characterized by the progressive loss of memory that may lead to inattentions and inability to focus at a task, language problems and behavioral changes.

Patients with Alzheimer's disease for instance may initially find themselves at a loss for words or unable to remember some bits of facts that happened the day before. But as the days progress, they will find themselves starting to forget important things like their addresses, their age and sometimes even their names.

Patients who are in the later stages of Alzheimer's will start to forget how to do routine things like brushing their teeth, taking a bath or using their utensils. Some may not speak altogether because they will often forget the words that they should be using or saying. Some will also behave differently, brought on by the frustration of not being able to do the things that they used to do. Often times, patients at the later stages will become dependents, acting like children who do not know what to do with themselves.

Although there are medicines that can slow down the progress of the disease especially if discovered early on, there is no solution to the problem. Once it settles into the system, it would be there for life and there is no chance of it ever disappearing.

Like medicines, there are activities that according to scientists can slow down the progression. Below are just some of them:

Read

Something as simple as reading the newspaper every day and keeping your mind informed with the latest news is already something that can prevent the disease from settling in. Just make it a point to use your brain. Be an analytical reader and raise questions and do not just absorb the texts and then forget about it. Being an active reader and allowing your imagination free reign will go a long way for exercising the brain. In fact, studies have shown that people who love to read are less likely to be diagnosed with Alzheimer's.

Answer Puzzles

Another mental exercise that people with Alzheimer's do to help slow down the process is to answer puzzles such as word hunts, cross words and even Sudoku. The more that you use your brain, the better will be your prognosis. Answering word games will also make sure that you practice words and increase your vocabulary, making it less likely for you to forget words and language.

Attend Classes

Being old does not mean that you cannot learn. Patients with Alzheimer's should make it a point to learn something new. This will exercise their brains. Creative tasks such as arts and crafts are another way to tap into the brain's resources without tiring them out. Learning a new thing also gives people with Alzheimer's the sense of purpose that they have lost since they were diagnosed with the disease.

www.ingramcontent.com/pod-product-compliance
Lightning Source LLC
Chambersburg PA
CBHW072342290526
45794CB00002B/984